Praise for The Green Food Diet

"I had no idea that the food we eat has been stripped of so many of its nutrients. It's shocking! So grateful for the practical steps this book gives for fixing that."

Samantha Murray – Olympic Silver medalist Modern Pentathlon London 2012 and World Champion 2014

"This is truly eye opening. To say we've been let down by Governments, supermarkets and the farming industry is an understatement. It's time to reclaim our health and the quality of our food."

James McDonald, BSc, Dip ION, ND – Sports Nutrition advisor for Team Tyco BMW and Moto GP

"The power of green foods to restore health and balance to our bodies and allow us to naturally help manage weight is incredible. This book really brings home the importance and the simplicity of how to restore that balance."

Professor Greg Whyte OBE, PhD, DSc, FBASES, FACSM

"The link between a healthy diet, a healthy active lifestyle and a healthy weight is becoming increasingly recognised by society as more and more scientific research is done on the subject. This is a very timely and powerful book."

Dr Nicola J Rowley, BSc, MPhil, PhD – Exercise Physiologist

"Humans have been unwittingly eliminating the most important nutrients from their diets for 10,000 years. And like every single person I've asked since reading this book I had no idea! Luckily I now know what to do about it."

Claire Forbes – Podiatrist, Jersey Channel Islands

"Unfortunately the nutrient levels in our food aren't anywhere near what they were like when Popeye was enjoying his Spinach; modern farming methods have removed so much of the goodness. That's why it's essential that we look to green superfoods as a staple part of our nutrition in order to provide us with the nutritional goodness we need at a cellular level."

Gemma Dawkins BSc, PGc – Nutrition Coach, Blogger

"It turns out that our hunter gatherer ancestors had a lot more high quality nutrition in their diets than we do. We, on the other hand, have a lot less nutrition and a lot more empty calories in our diet and that's why so many of us are unhealthy and overweight. The Green Food Diet shows us how we can easily fix that, lose weight and get healthy. This is a very important book."

Dr Larry Milam – Vice President of the University of Natural Medicine California

"Who would have imagined that there are potatoes 28 times more nutritious than the ones we normally eat... only we can't buy them, because the supermarkets won't sell them to us."

Andy Mackenzie – Performance Director Pentathlon Ireland

THE
GREEN FOOD
DIET

Avoid the Hidden Dangers
in Your Food and Eat Your Way
to Vibrant Health
and Your Perfect Weight

James Greenwell

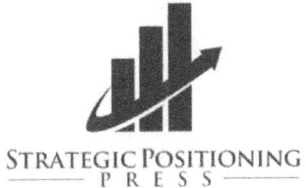

STRATEGIC POSITIONING
——— P R E S S ———

Oxford and Bath

THE GREEN FOOD DIET

Published by Strategic Positioning Press Limited

Printed by CreateSpace
1st edition

First published in 2017

ISBN-13: 978-1508523215
ISBN-10: 1508523215

Strategic Positioning Press Limited
Unit 5
Brook Lane
Westbury
Wiltshire, BA13 4ES
United Kingdom

Disclaimer

The information contained in this book is the opinion of the author and is intended for educational purposes only. The author is not a medical doctor and the information contained in this book does not constitute medical advice of any kind. This book is made available with the understanding that author is not giving medical advice of any kind and that neither the book nor the dietary information or suggestions within the book are intended to replace medical advice, or to diagnose, prescribe or treat any disease, condition, illness or injury, whether physical or psychological. You are responsible for your own health and well-being and you should consult a licensed physician and receive medical clearance before starting any new diet, weight loss program or exercise program including anything contained in this book. If you plan to commence an exercise program then you should also get advice from an appropriately qualified exercise professional before doing so.

The author and the publisher specifically disclaim any liability, damage, loss or risk, personal or otherwise, caused or alleged to be caused as a consequence, directly or indirectly, of the use, application or interpretation of any of the information contained within this book.

No governmental or medical authorities have evaluated the information contained within this book.

"Let food be thy medicine and let medicine be thy food."

—Hippocrates (c. 460 BC – 370 BC)

Contents

The Green Food Diet

Avoid the Hidden Dangers in Your Food and Eat Your Way to Vibrant Health and Your Perfect Weight

This book will help you lose weight.

And if you're already at a healthy weight it will help you maintain it.

However, it's not a diet book in the traditional sense and it's about much more than just weight loss. It's about avoiding the hidden dangers of our modern diet and replacing bad foods with the foods we need for health, energy, vitality and disease prevention.

Our bodies possess incredible powers of repair and regeneration. But they can only work with the building blocks we give them. A healthy body is impossible without a healthy diet.

This book will help you get both.

Why do we spend so much time dieting?

A recent UK study of 2,000 people found that three quarters of men and women had tried at least one diet in the last year. And, amazingly, it found that by the age of 45 the average woman had tried 61 different diets!

Unfortunately, an estimated 80% of people who manage to actually lose weight gain some or all of it back within a year.

Even more worryingly, 35% of dieters actually gain back more weight than they lost in the first place.

Clearly most diets are not working or we wouldn't have to keep starting new ones. But why is that? And what can we do to fix it?

How can we make weight loss easy instead of difficult? How can we end the cycle of struggling to lose a few pounds only to gain them back within a few weeks?

The good news is that losing weight really doesn't have to be that hard. But it has to be based on the way our bodies actually work and not on the latest diet fad or gimmick. And, of course, that success has to be long-term: the weight we lose has to stay off for good.

This short book will show you how it's possible to lose weight quickly, easily and permanently with just a few simple changes to your diet.

It's based on our scientific understanding of how our bodies really work and what we need to do to lose weight and keep it off successfully:

> A successful diet should be healthy and include a wide variety of nutrients – too many faddy diets sacrifice health and nutrition in search of the latest quick fix.

> A successful diet must be easy to follow for as long as it takes you to lose the desired amount of weight. In other words, you should never find yourself feeling hungry.

> It must be effective at stimulating weight loss. Many diets have the opposite effect – they cause the metabolism to actually slow down.

> The results must be long-term: a diet is not successful if you end up piling the pounds back on as soon as the diet stops.

Well, here's the good news: such a diet exists. It's easy to do, easy to stick to, healthy and the results are amazing. People who have struggled for years to lose weight and all but given up hope have been able to lose weight rapidly on this diet *and* keep it off!

It's very common for people to enjoy consistent weight loss of two pounds a week or more. This may not sound like a huge amount, but it starts to add up very quickly. It means 20 pounds of weight loss every 10 weeks.

And – because the diet is easy to stick to and the results come quickly and consistently – it's easy to stay motivated, since we get motivation from a sense of progress and success.

Meanwhile, because it's designed to make sure that you don't ever feel hungry it doesn't rely on our finite supply of willpower. In fact, you may well find that you are actually eating *more* than you're used to!

Many diets founder on the rocks of temptation: when the dieter's willpower is no longer strong enough to steer them away from the foods they know will wreck their diet. Scientific studies prove that – when it comes to dieting – our willpower is at its lowest when we are hungry. By taking hunger, and therefore willpower, out of the equation we make the weight loss process much easier, much more likely to succeed and turn it into a much more enjoyable process.

There's one thing about the Green Food Diet that's so important I want to say it again before we move on: *you should never feel hungry while you are on it.* If you feel hungry then you're doing it wrong!

The reason the Green Food Diet is so successful is because it is based on *adding* healthy and nutritious foods to your diet rather than on taking foods away. Again, scientific studies prove that from a psychological point of view this is a much more successful approach to weight loss.

That's because the moment we start telling ourselves that we can't have something it becomes a temptation – a forbidden food. If instead we focus on consuming more of the healthy, nutrient rich foods that we know promote weight loss then things feel very different. It's no longer about abstinence, denial and temptation. Instead, we have a *positive* focus: trying to eat *more* of foods that we know are good for us.

What are the best weight loss foods and why?

The best weight loss foods are vegetables, salad, beans, pulses, legumes and fruits (there are a lot of myths currently going around about fruit and fructose – I'll deal with these later on). Of these foods the best – in terms of weight loss – are green vegetables, particularly green leafy vegetables.

The more of these foods we can add to our diet the more weight we will lose and the faster that weight will come off.

There are several reasons why these foods are so good at promoting weight loss. Most importantly, are very low in calories. Much lower, gram for gram, than most of the other foods we normally eat. This means that they have a powerful "displacement effect." In other words, the more fruit and veg we eat the less of the other – much more calorically dense – foods we eat. These "saved" calories start to add up very quickly and the more we displace the quicker we will lose weight.

By the way, much of the time I'll be using "fruit and veg" as shorthand for fruit, vegetables, salad vegetables, beans, pulses and legumes. As you can see, it's a bit less of a mouthful!

Fruit and veg also happen to be very filling, which helps keep our overall food intake down without us feeling hungry. This is partly because they are rich in dietary fibre, which promotes satiety – the feeling that we have had enough to eat. The fibre in fruits and vegetables has all sorts of other health and weight loss benefits as well, which we'll come back to later.

Fruits and vegetables prevent disease

Over the last few decades an overwhelming body of research has shown that eating more fruit and veg has a protective effect against a whole range of serious diseases. These include heart disease, high blood pressure (hypertension), stroke, cancer, diabetes and pulmonary (lung) disease.

Conversely, a low intake of fruit and veg correlates with an increased likelihood of being overweight or obese. And being overweight has the opposite effect – it increases our chances of getting all of these life threatening diseases.

But that's not the worst part: the worst part is that these diseases come as a package. Heart disease, high blood pressure, increased risk of stroke and increased cancer risk are pretty much guaranteed if you are overweight. Diabetes takes longer to develop, but if the underlying weight problems persist for long enough then it too is all but guaranteed: Being overweight is the single biggest risk factor for diabetes, as demonstrated by the fact that 85 percent of diabetics are overweight.

And diabetes is serious – a lot more serious than most people realise. There's a reason it's known as "the silent killer"...

it is a cause of heart disease in its own right

it is the leading cause of blindness in the West

it is the leading cause of kidney failure

it is the leading cause of limb amputations

it causes high blood pressure

it is a major cause of nerve damage (neuropathy)

it significantly increases the risk of certain types of cancer

This cocktail of risk factors leads to a significant reduction in quality of life with increased risk of an early death. In 2007 diabetes was officially linked to 231,404 deaths in the United States alone, while in the UK – according to figures from the 2011 National Diabetes Audit – around 1 death in 20 is caused by diabetes. In fact, the true figures are probably much higher as very often diabetes is a contributing causal factor that goes unreported.

This is all very sad, but there is lots of good news:

1) Type 2 diabetes is one of the most preventable diseases there is. According to the Harvard School of Public Health (HSPH), studies have shown that not smoking, eating a healthy diet, and keeping a healthy weight (a body mass index of under 25) reduces the risk of diabetes by 90 percent.

Type 2 diabetes is not just preventable – it is in fact reversible. Research has shown that by restricting their calorie intake and losing sufficient body fat type 2 diabetics can not only reverse their diabetes, they can then stay diabetes free. This is true even in the case of diabetics who have had the condition for years.

2) By increasing our intake of fruit and veg we can also dramatically reduce our risk of heart disease, high blood pressure, stroke, cancer, diabetes and pulmonary disease.

3) Increased fruit and veg intake also helps prevent osteoporosis and age related eye disease – in particular, cataracts and AMD (age related macular degeneration).

4) By increasing our intake of fruit and veg we can quickly begin to get down to a healthy weight. Apart from being a great goal in itself, maintaining a healthy weight significantly reduces our risk of all of these killer diseases.

It's clear that the common denominator to achieving all these benefits is increasing the amount of fruit and veg that we eat.

Let's take a moment to look at why eating fruit and veg is so beneficial to both our health and our weight loss efforts. I think it's important to understand why this is because having that understanding will give you the belief and motivation you need to succeed: My experience with countless clients over the years is that – to paraphrase Oprah Winfrey – "when people know better they do better".

We are "the most overfed and undernourished generation in history"

Because of the abundance of cheap, heavily processed convenience food that is now available we have been described as "the most overfed and undernourished generation in history." In other words, most of us get far too many calories and not nearly enough quality nutrition.

Even supposedly healthy foods – such as most cereal products – are stripped of much of the nutrition that they once contained. Partly this is the result of modern intensive farming methods – for example, fertilisers add nitrogen to soil but cause other important minerals to be leached away. Partly this is because foods are often deliberately stripped of key nutrients during processing, either to improve their flavour or to increase their shelf life. There are other reasons, but we'll come back to those later.

In order to properly understand what a *healthy* diet should contain it is necessary to understand the difference between macro-nutrients and micro-nutrients. Quite simply, macro-nutrients are what we would consider to be the main food groups: carbohydrates, proteins and fats. Macro-nutrients provide us with the energy we need to carry out our daily activities. Micro-nutrients are vitamins, minerals and other nutrients that we require in very small quantities to maintain good health. In order to ensure that we get a sufficient range and quantity of micro-nutrients in our diet we must make sure that the macro-nutrients – or energy foods – that we eat are chosen from a wide range of healthy sources.

As described above, the typical Western diet contains too many energy rich macro-nutrients and too few micro-nutrients. This, of course, has adverse health consequences.

Conversely, a healthy diet will include a wide range of food sources that promote optimum health. This goal is achieved by including a range of 'powerhouse' foods that are packed full of the nutrients we need: in particular, fruits and vegetables that are rich in vitamins, minerals, antioxidants, phyto-chemicals, enzymes and fibre (fibre is not technically a nutrient, but is very important nonetheless).

So how much fruit and veg do we need?

It's clear that eating plenty of fruit and veg helps us to lose weight (and keep it off) as well as having huge health benefits, but how much should we be eating?

The truth about 5-a-day

I'm sure you've heard about getting your "5-a-day."

It was a useful campaign to get people to think about and increase their daily intake of fruit and veg. However, it turns out that the Government wasn't being entirely honest with us – no great surprise there then!

Even before it ran the campaign the Government knew full well that 5 servings of fruit and veg a day was well short of the optimum amount needed for good health.

So why did they run the campaign? Well, at the time the average person was eating so little fruit and veg the Government felt that setting the target any higher than 5-a-day would be so unrealistic for most people that it would put them off from even trying.

In other words, they were coming from the right place in terms of trying to improve people's eating habits. But by running the campaign they did they have misled millions of people into thinking that 5-a-day is all they need – whereas, in fact, 5-a-day is really the bare minimum.

Before we go on, what is a serving?

First of all, what is a serving?

You'll see all sorts of examples of serving sizes, most of which I don't think are entirely helpful. A serving is "a medium this" or "a small that" or a "large such and such". Or it's a handful of something (whose hand one wonders?). Or it's a cup... or half a cup. It's as if people are trying to make things as confusing as possible!

Fortunately, there is an "official" serving size based on weight. And while it may not always be convenient to weigh things, once you've don't it a few times you'll have a good visual picture of what a serving is and you can stop worrying about the scales.

The simple answer is that a serving is 80 grams or 3 ounces of fruit, vegetables, salad, beans, pulses or legumes – easy enough so far. It gets a bit more complicated in the case of dried fruit and fruit juices or smoothies.

With dried fruit the nutrition is more concentrated – on a weight for weight basis – since much of the water has been taken out. Because of this you only need about 30 grams of dried fruit to make up one serving. However, if you are trying to lose weight I recommend staying away from dried fruit as much as you can, since as well as concentrating the good nutrition (antioxidants, phyto-chemicals, etc.) the drying process also concentrates the bad nutrition – i.e., the sugars.

In the case of fruit juice and smoothies around 150 ml (5 fluid ounces) normally counts as one serving. However, as with dried fruit I recommend that you try to avoid fruit juice and smoothies if you are trying to lose weight. Juiced fruits are much less filling than whole fruits, since you digest them much faster. Faster digestion also means that the sugars they contain will enter your blood stream much faster. Both these things are bad news if you are trying to lose weight and so the best thing is to avoid them altogether.

So how much fruit and veg should we be eating?

It turns out, rather confusingly, that there are lots of different recommendations out there. The current UK official recommendation is 5-a-day, but we've already seen that this number is not based on what is optimum for our health. There are studies recommending 7 servings, 8 servings, 9 servings, 13 servings, 14 servings and more per day.

Perhaps more usefully, some of the more recent guidelines advocate increasing the amount of fruit and veg you eat in line with the number of calories you consume. This makes sense since someone needing 3,000 calories a day to maintain their weight will – all other things being equal – require more nutritional support to stay healthy than someone who only needs to consume 2,000 calories a day.

The 2005 Dietary Guidelines for Americans recommend 9 servings per day for someone on 2,000 calories a day. This equates to 13½ servings for someone eating 3,000 calories a day.

These guidelines are much more useful than the traditional 5-a-day mantra (which has now been officially dropped in the US, though it persists in the UK).

Bear in mind, however, that these recommendations are based on what is required for a healthy diet – not on what is needed for healthy, rapid and sustainable weight loss.

When you're trying to lose weight the more fruit and veg you can eat better! Of course, you still need an adequate intake of protein and healthy fats, but it's the fruit and veg that are really going to turbo-charge your success.

How to lose weight by eating more!

I know I mentioned this earlier, but it's important enough to say again: For all the reasons we've already discussed, *adding* the right kinds of foods to your diet (more fruit, veg, salad, beans, pulses and legumes) is the single most effective strategy when it comes to fast, successful and long-term weight loss.

Eating lots of these foods will – due to the "displacement effect" – lead naturally and effortlessly to you eating less of other more calorically dense foods. The result is that your excess weight will quickly start to melt away and your health will improve.

9 simple steps for you to follow

Dieting should not be difficult, complicated or stressful!

Here are some simple steps that will help you dramatically increase the amount of fruit and veg you eat so that you can begin losing weight fast.

1) Go for variety! Try lots of different fruits, vegetables, salad vegetables, beans, pulses and legumes so that your diet stays interesting. Try them in combination with one another to increase the variety.

2) Convenience is crucial! Shop, plan and prepare ahead of time so that you have fruit and veg available when you need it. If you're out and about all day what strategies can you put in place ahead of time to make sure you have fruit and veg with you when you need to eat?

3) Visibility is key – especially to start with. Put fruit and crudités where you can see them so that you'll be reminded to eat more. Having a fruit bowl in my office has been a big help in boosting the amount I eat as it combines convenience *and* visibility.

4) Every meal, every day! If you can get into the habit of having some fruit and/or veg with every meal you will be able to dramatically increase your overall intake and be making a huge step towards losing weight.

5) Snack on fruit, snack on veg. Not only will this help to stop you from ever feeling hungry (remember, you should never feel hungry on this diet), it will also help to increase your overall intake and speed up your weight loss. This is where the fruit bowl and the crudités really help.

6) Half a plate... or more: for lunch and dinner try to make sure that at least half your plate is covered with vegetables or salad (it can be more!).

7) If you're still feeling hungry keep going! If you've finished your meal and you still feel hungry then top up on more veg or snack on some fruit – all completely guilt free!

8) Track your servings – at least to begin with. It's true that "what we measure we manage" and so it's important to track how much fruit and veg you're eating for at least the first week or two until you have established some good habits. Remember, 80 grams or 3 ounces equals one serving. How many servings did you have today?

9) Develop good habits: If you want to see what your future looks like then look at your habits today – and if you don't like what you see then you'll need to choose some better habits. All of the steps I've mentioned above can be turned into habits. It might take anything from a few days up to a month, but it will happen if you stick with it – and the more habitual things become the easier they are.

Additional guidelines

Here are some additional guidelines that will help you get the most out of the 9 steps above.

1) Try to hit at least 10 servings a day. Whatever your calorie intake, I recommend aiming for at least 10 servings a day – it's not as hard as it sounds if you follow the 9 steps above.

2) If you can eat more than 10 then do so... and give yourself a big pat on the back!

3) Limit your fruit intake to 4 servings a day (whatever your total intake). A range of studies clearly show that people who eat more fruit weight less – despite all the recent alarm about fructose. However, you still don't want too much fructose in your diet so limit yourself to 4 servings of fruit a day and get the rest of your intake from veg, salad, beans, pulses and legumes.

4) The greener the better! The more green leafy vegetables and cruciferous vegetables you can eat the better – these are the Kings and Queens of weight loss! They are packed with nutrients, high in fibre, very filling and low in calories – the perfect weight loss combination.

In my opinion, the Top Gun of weight loss vegetables – "the best of the best" – is spinach, but here's a list of other great green leafy and cruciferous veg:

Broccoli

Cauliflower

Cabbage

Brussels sprouts

Broccoli romanesco

Bok choy

Pak choy

Spinach

Kale

Spring greens

Collard greens

Chard

Watercress

Seaweed

5) Potatoes don't count :-(Sorry, but potatoes are packed with carbs and they aren't going to help you lose weight. Sweet potatoes are a better choice – they are slower digesting and extremely rich in beta-carotene. However, the more you can cut down your intake of starchy carbs (potatoes, sweet potatoes, rice, bread, cereals and pasta) the faster you will lose weight.

As alternatives to potatoes try turnips, parsnips, swedes and squashes, all of which can be mashed or roasted. Cauliflower can also be used as a substitute for mashed potatoes.

6) Beans, pulses and legumes are basically interchangeable terms, but I've been using all three to make sure we're not leaving anything out. They are a great slow digesting, high fibre and high protein addition to your diet. However, I recommend you stay away from the baked beans because of the added sugar they contain.

7) Go easy on the dressing. Salad is great – you can eat as much as you want and it's ridiculously low in calories! Just go easy on the dressing. Most salad dressings are oil based and so high in calories, yet there are plenty of healthy alternatives. You could try salsa, hummus, cottage cheese, balsamic vinegar, lemon or lime, salt and pepper, nuts and seeds, as well as experimenting with herbs and spices. Make sure you have plenty of variety so you don't get bored.

8) Remember to avoid fruit juice and smoothies while you're trying to lose weight – they digest quickly and contain lots of sugars and so promote weight gain.

When you combine these guidelines with the 9 steps above you'll be able to develop some fantastic healthy eating habits and dramatically boost your intake of fruit and veg. As a result you'll quickly start losing weight. Plus, you will boost your general health, wellbeing and vitality as well as reducing your risk of heart disease, high blood pressure, stroke, cancer, diabetes, pulmonary disease, aged related eye disease and osteoporosis.

And best of all, it's not a diet! At least it's not a diet in the sense that we normally think of them.

Instead, it's a simple and easy to follow <u>healthy eating plan</u>.

And, most important of all, unlike normal diets it's not about denial and forced abstinence – instead, it's about adding a range of healthy and wholesome foods to your diet. No more calorie counting and no more feeling miserable and hungry the whole time!

A word of warning...

There is, unfortunately, a catch – something you need to know before you start – though it has nothing to do with the diet itself.

And the catch is that our fruit and veg is not as nutritious as it once was – not even close. I'll explain why this is and what you can do about it in a moment, but, essentially, the issue is connected to the problem we were talking about earlier: that we are the most overfed and undernourished generation in history.

This is something urgently needs fixing, but it's something we're going to have to do for ourselves at an individual level. It's not something that the farming or food industries are going to be doing any time soon and you certainly shouldn't be waiting for any help from governments!

You would think that your fruits and veggies today are the same as the fruits and veggies from ten or twenty or fifty years ago, but they're not. The level of micro-nutrients they contain is falling every year – and it is the micro-nutrients that provide us with all the important health benefits we've been talking about.

The fact is, fruit and vegetables today are lower in vitamins, minerals, phyto-chemicals and antioxidants than at any time in history, and it is our health that is suffering as a result.

Evidence for this comes from a whole range of studies looking at the decline in nutrient content of various fruits and vegetables over the last 50 to 100 years.

The numbers are shocking!

Let me give you some examples from different studies:

Broccoli that has lost 75% of its calcium

Carrots that have lost 75% of their magnesium

Watercress that has lost 88% of its iron

Apples that have lost 85% of their phosphorous

Spinach that has lost 59% of its vitamin C

Peaches that have lost 96% of their vitamin A

To put these numbers in perspective, they mean that based on these studies you would have to eat four times as much broccoli today to get the same amount of calcium as before. And if you think that is bad, consider having to eat 25 peaches to get the same amount of vitamin A as you would have got from *a single peach* in the past!

Incredible declines like this can be found in study after study and for all kinds of fruits and vegetables.

Before we go on there are some important points to note about the nutritional state of our fruit and veg today:

First, the declines are not limited to the vitamins and minerals listed above – they apply to the full spectrum of vitamins and minerals, as well as phyto-chemicals and antioxidants. So for example, broccoli has not only lost up to 75% of its calcium, it has also lost significant amounts of vitamins E, thiamine (vitamin B1), riboflavin (vitamin B2), pantothenic acid (vitamin B5), iron, magnesium, phosphorus and selenium – as well as a whole range of phyto-chemicals and antioxidants.

Second, these declines are not limited just to the fruits and vegetables listed above – they apply to all the fruits, vegetables, salad vegetables, beans, pulses and legumes (and this is happening worldwide).

Third, not all of the declines are as dramatic as the ones listed above – for example, not all peaches have lost 96% of their vitamin A. There are numerous factors that influence the extent of nutrient depletion, as we shall see in a moment. However, very significant declines have taken place across the board, with vitamin and mineral levels in most non-organic crops having dropped by between 20% and 75% over the course of the last century.

Something else to bear in mind is that in our modern world our bodies have to cope with both levels *and* varieties of toxins, pollutants and environmental chemicals that are unprecedented in human history. To cope with the biological stress these cause and to detoxify our systems we need more micro-nutrients, not less. The decline in the nutritional quality of our food could not be coming at a worse time.

Governments have known about this for decades...

This is not a new phenomenon – it is simply one that has got worse over time and which seems to be accelerating. Here is an incriminating extract from an official document published for the US Senate:

> *...countless human ills stem from the fact that [the] impoverished soil of America no longer provides plant foods with the mineral elements essential to human nourishment and health.*
>
> *Do you know that most of us today are suffering from certain dangerous diet deficiencies which cannot be remedied until the depleted soils from which our foods come are brought into proper mineral balance?*
>
> *And the alarming fact is that foods—fruits and vegetables and grains—now being raised on millions of acres of land that no longer contains enough of certain needed minerals, are starving us—no matter how much of them we eat!*

Would you believe that this document was published in **June 1936** and yet today, nearly 80 years later, few people – whether in the US, the UK or anywhere else in the world – are aware of the problem!

Rex Beach, the author of the report, ends it with a question that is both profound and prophetic: *"It is simpler to cure sick soils than sick people—which shall we choose?"*

What a shame that governments, supermarkets and big agro-business either don't agree with him or don't care enough to do anything about it.

That is why it's so important we take control of the problem ourselves – at an individual level. Actions speak louder than words and the people we've assumed are safeguarding the quality of our food have proved – over the course of many decades – that they cannot be trusted with the job. If we wait for them to make the necessary changes we will be waiting somewhere between a very long time and forever!

What is causing this terrible decline?

Worryingly (because it makes it a lot harder to fix the problem), there are lots of reasons why the nutrient levels in our foods are declining so seriously – some or all of which affect *all* of the non-organic shop bought fruits and vegetables we eat. In fact, even organic produce is not immune to the problem, although it is generally a much better – if more expensive – alternative.

Here are some of the reasons why the nutrition content of our fruit and veg has deteriorated so badly over the last century:

1) The "dilution effect" – the dilution effect is caused by an increase in the weight of a crop, which leads to a decrease in the concentration of minerals and other nutrients it contains.

It is caused by various intensive farming methods designed to increase crop yields, such as the heavy use of fertilisers. These methods cause crops to grow faster than is natural and as a result they are unable to take up enough micronutrients to maintain normal concentrations.

2) The "genetic dilution effect" – the genetic dilution affect is similar in its results to the dilution effect, the difference being that it is caused by the selection of crops for their yield – either through genetic engineering or simply through the progressive selection of varieties that produce bigger yields.

Of course, the yields being selected for are size, weight and carbohydrate levels – not the health giving micronutrient and phyto-chemical levels.

3) "Unbalanced" plants – we are now seeing "unbalanced" plants with root systems that are too shallow for their size. This is because they have been progressively chosen on the basis of yield, which over time tends to lead to the selection of plants that put more energy into the valuable fruit, vegetable or grain and less energy into their root system.

This exacerbates the dilution effects described above, because the plants are left with a root system that is insufficient for their micro-nutritional needs (excessive fertiliser use is what enables them to grow despite their poor root systems).

4) Over farming – agricultural land is now more intensively farmed than at any time in human history. Crops are not properly rotated, land is not left fallow, soil nutrients are not replenished – even the *spacing* between plants is much closer!

As a result, soil is being depleted of its nutrients far faster than they can be replenished. Over farming is also causing the erosion of topsoil and the depletion of important bacterial communities within the soil that remains.

5) Transportation – years ago fresh produce was much more likely to be consumed locally that is today when journeys of hundreds or thousands of miles are common and our food can often come from a different continent.

Because it can take several days for produce to reach the shops it is often picked before it is fully ripe meaning that it doesn't have the chance to develop fully, thus compromising its micro-nutrient content. Meanwhile, light, heat and oxygen have much more time to degrade the vitamin, enzyme and antioxidant content of the produce, with as much as half being lost.

6) Excessive use of fertilisers – as well as contributing to the dilution effect, fertilisers cause two other significant problems: The first is that they can interfere with the ability of plants to absorb nutrients from the soil. The second is that they leach minerals from the soil. The leached minerals are then washed away by rainwater further degrading the soil.

7) Excessive use of pesticides, herbicides and fungicides – pesticides, herbicides and fungicides can interfere with a plant's ability to absorb nutrients. They can also damage or destroy certain nutrients either before can be absorbed or even within the plant itself. They too can cause minerals to Leach from the soil – further impoverishing soil quality.

8) Selection for taste – fruits and vegetables have long been selected for taste, both to reduce bitterness and fibre content and to increase sweetness. Unfortunately, many of the most beneficial phyto-nutrients in plants have a bitter taste. Conversely, sweeter produce contains more sugars, which tends to reduce the concentration of the all-important micro-nutrients.

All of these issues contribute to the huge scale of the problem facing us today. In a moment, we'll look at the steps we can take to protect ourselves from the dangerous decline in the nutrition content of our fruit and veg.

A historical footnote that is both interesting and alarming is that, while things have got much worse over the last century, the problem of declining nutrient levels in our food is not new. It actually began 10,000 years ago with the dawn of agricultural history: This was when we first began to domesticate wild plants and, of course, when we first began selecting for taste.

Researchers have been able to compare the phyto-nutrient content of the sorts of wild plants that our hunter gatherer ancestors would have eaten with those in our modern supermarkets. The results are truly shocking.

In a recent article, published in the New York Times, author Jo Robinson gave the following examples:

Wild dandelions, once a springtime treat for Native Americans, have seven times more phyto-nutrients than spinach, which we consider a "superfood." A purple potato native to Peru has 28 times more cancer-fighting anthocyanins than common russet potatoes. One species of apple has a staggering 100 times more phyto-nutrients than the Golden Delicious displayed in our supermarkets.

The implications of this are huge. It means things may be even worse than we thought. You see nearly all of the studies into the declining nutrition levels in our foods have looked at them over relatively short time horizons – usually just the last few decades, as opposed to the last 10,000 years!

Think for a moment about the last example cited above: an apple that has 100 times more phyto-nutrients than a Golden Delicious. Now imagine similar examples across the board, with all your fruits and vegetables giving you no more than a tiny fraction of the nutrients found in their wild ancestors.

It is no wonder that we are the most over fed and under nourished generation in history, with all the health risks that that entails.

What can you do about it?

Here are some suggestions as to what you can do to try and get optimum levels of nutrition from your fruit and veg:

1) Eat more fruit and veg – this may seem obvious, but it is critical if we are to get enough nutrition for optimum health. If the fruit and veg we eat is deficient in nutrients then we need to make a special effort to eat more of it to make up for the nutritional shortfall.

2) Eat organic – eating organic does not solve all of these problems; however, (and despite strident claims to the contrary from the non-organic food lobby) the micro-nutrient levels in organic produce tend to be *significantly* higher than those found in their intensively farmed non-organic counterparts. The downside to eating organic is that it can be more expensive.

3) Buying local – buying more of your produce locally – for example, from farmers' markets – reduces the problems associated with long transportation times and the resulting deterioration in nutrient levels.

4) Buy before you eat – it may not always be convenient, but if you can then buy your fruit and veg close to the time when you are going to eat it. The fresher it is the more nutrients will remain.

5) Store carefully – once you have bought your produce store it somewhere that is cool or refrigerated and which is dark.

6) Eat raw – fruits, salad vegetables, crudités and some vegetables can be eaten raw. This helps to preserve both the enzyme and the vitamin content.

7) Lightly cook your vegetables – just to confuse matters, some vegetables are better for you if they are cooked rather than eaten raw. Tomatoes are a classic example as cooking them dramatically increases the bioavailability of the important cancer fighting antioxidant lycopene.

However you choose to cook your vegetables you're generally better off if you go easy on them – lightly steaming them or gently stir frying them so that they still retain plenty of crunch are good options. Boiling is, in most cases, the least healthy option.

8) Seek out dark colours – the rule of thumb is that the darker the colour of a fruit or vegetable the more phyto-nutrients it contains. And if that colour extends all the way through the plant rather than being just skin deep then even better.

9) Grow your own – again, this will not be possible for everyone, but if you can why not think about growing your own fruits, vegetables and salad plants? This gives you complete control over the entire process, including which varieties you choose, what goes into the soil and what, if anything, goes on to the plants.

The more of these suggestions you can follow the better. Unfortunately, for most of us it still won't be enough to guarantee optimum health. Even if you organically grow all of your own produce it will still be difficult – if not impossible – to find varieties that are as nutrient dense as their wild ancestors were before we started selecting for taste all those thousands of years ago.

So if we still can't get the level of nutrition we truly need from our fruit and veg is there anything else we can do?

There is good news...

The good news is that there is something we can do about it.

In fact, it's actually possible to supercharge our nutrient intake to the point that the micro-nutrient levels in our diet rival or even surpass those we could get from the pre-domesticated fruits and vegetables that were available to our hunter-gatherer ancestors 10,000 years ago.

The way we do this is by adding to our diet certain specially selected and naturally occurring green foods that are incredibly nutrient rich. Not only are these green foods organic, they are essentially unchanged from their wild ancestors. As a result, they are still packed with the same micro-nutrients that they would have contained thousands or even tens of thousands of years ago. This makes them far more "nutritionally dense" than the foods that we normally eat.

By eating these specially selected green-foods we can make up for the micro-nutrient shortfall in our fruit and veg.

Now just to be clear, I am not saying that we should eat these green-foods *instead* of fruit and veg. I am saying we should be eating them *as well as* having lots of fruit and veg (ideally the 10 or more servings a day that I talked about earlier).

I first began supplementing my diet with green superfoods like these nineteen years ago and was so impressed by the results that I've been eating them ever since. I still eat lots of fruit and veg as well, but I think of these green superfoods as my "insurance" policy. They guarantee that I get an outstanding level of nutrition every day, regardless of any shortcomings in the other foods I eat.

The way I get my green superfoods is by taking a supplement called Green Magic. Green Magic is a blend of 17 different nutrient dense foods, 8 of which are green superfoods together with 9 other foods all of which have key health benefits.

Because the foods it contains are so nutrient dense, Green Magic is extremely rich in vitamins, minerals, antioxidants, phyto-chemicals, enzymes, amino acids, essential fatty acids and soluble fibre.

Taking antioxidants as an example will give you an idea of just how nutrient rich Green Magic is:

The antioxidant activity of foods can be measured by what is known as the ORAC scale (ORAC stands for Oxygen Radical Absorbance Capacity). The higher a food's ORAC score the more antioxidants it contains.

One 3 gram serving of Green Magic (a rounded teaspoon) contains 1,839 ORAC units – that's the equivalent ORAC value of 5 typical servings of fruit and veg. In other words, despite being only 12 calories, one serving of Green Magic gives you the same antioxidant benefits as the traditional 5-a-day!

Green Magic is about much more than antioxidants, however. The 17 different foods in Green Magic contain a wide variety of healthy nutrients and micro-nutrients. Here are the ingredients of Green Magic, together with some of the key nutrients they contain:

The 8 green superfoods

Hawaiian Spirulina – Spirulina is a blue-green algae. It is the world's richest natural source of plant protein and contains all the essential amino acids. It is also a rich source of iron and is packed with vitamins, minerals, enzymes, antioxidants and phyto-chemicals.

Chlorella – Chlorella is a green algae. As the world's richest source of chlorophyll it has a powerful detoxifying effect on the body. It is particularly rich in beta carotene.

Wheat Grass Juice – Taken from the young fresh shoots, wheat grass juice is rich in enzymes and chlorophyll. It is also a great source of vitamin E, several B vitamins, manganese and zinc. (An important side note – Wheat Grass Juice is gluten free since it comes from the leaf shoots and *not* the grain.)

Barley Grass Juice – Another juice rich in enzymes and chlorophyll, barley grass juice is also a rich source of potassium, calcium and iron. (Again, Barley Grass Juice is gluten free since it is from the grass *not* the grain.)

Kamut Juice – Kamut is an ancient Egyptian wheat, unchanged for at least four thousand years. Kamut juice is taken from the plant's new shoots, rather than the grain, and so is gluten free. It has a powerful alkalising and detoxifying effect on the body.

Icelandic Kelp – Icelandic kelp is a sea vegetable that is especially rich in minerals and trace-minerals. It is also a good source of fibre and vitamin K.

Nova Scotia Dulse – Another sea vegetable that is very rich in minerals and trace-minerals. It is a particularly good source of potassium and lithium.

Wheat Sprouts – Wheat sprouts are a great source of vitamins, minerals, enzymes and antioxidants and are rich in phosphorous (and are gluten free).

The 9 other key nutrients

Lecithin – Lecithin emulsifies fat and so is important for cardiovascular health. It is an important brain food and is high in choline, which helps us burn fat. Lecithin may also reduce bad (LDL) cholesterol levels and raise good (HDL) cholesterol levels.

High Pectin Apple Fibre – High pectin apple fibre is a soluble fibre that helps to trap cholesterol and remove it from the body. It reduces the risk of heart disease and improves digestive health.

Rice Kernel Membrane Powder – A great source of fibre, rice kernel membrane powder is also rich in B vitamins and vitamin E.

Superoxide Dismutase (SOD) and Catalase – Both are powerful antioxidant enzymes that reduce oxidative stress in the body, reduce inflammation and slow the aging process.

Co Enzyme Q10 (CoQ10) – As well as being a powerful antioxidant, CoQ10 is vital for energy production, the highest concentrations being found in our major organs. CoQ10 levels decline as we get older so supplementation is important for maintaining energy levels and vitality.

Royal Jelly – Royal jelly is a rich in antioxidants, enzymes and B vitamins. It also contains 22 amino acids including all the essential amino acids.

Jerusalem Artichoke Powder (JAP) – JAP is a prebiotic and an excellent source of fructooligosaccharides. As such it helps maintain the friendly bacteria in our gut and so promotes digestive health. It is rich in thiamine, iron, phosphorous and potassium and is a natural source of inulin.

Lactobacillus Acidophilus – Lactobacillus acidophilus is a probiotic (or "friendly" bacteria) that is vitally important for proper digestive health. It may also improve the body's immune response and help us maintain a healthy weight.

Bifidus Bacterium – Bifidus bacterium is another probiotic that is also vital for proper digestive health and which, again, may improve immune our function and help us maintain a healthy weight.

This is by no means an exhaustive list of the nutrients found in the 17 ingredients that Green Magic contains – just some highlights. But it's enough for you to be able to see why Green

Magic is such a powerful supplement. It is also dairy, lactose, gluten and GMO free.

The benefits of Green Magic

Because it contains such a wide spectrum of nutrients Green Magic is an amazingly complete supplement. Here are some of the key health benefits of Green Magic:

> **Weight loss** – Green Magic is not designed as a weight loss supplement – for example, it has no artificial stimulants such as caffeine or guarana. However, weight loss – or more specifically the loss of excess body fat – is one of the happy "side effects" of Green Magic.

This is because by improving digestive health and liver function (Green Magic has a detoxifying effect on the liver) Green Magic helps us lose excess weight naturally. An increasing number of studies are linking the importance of digestive health to maintaining a healthy weight. The enzymes, prebiotics, probiotics and soluble fibre in Green Magic all help to improve our digestive function and help us maintain a healthy weight.

A healthy liver, meanwhile, helps us maintain stable blood sugar levels. It is also able to do a much better job of utilising stored body fat and burning it for current energy needs.

Not only does this mean that we will tend to eat less (particularly less of the sort of unhealthy sugary and fatty snacks that are most likely to promote weight gain) it also makes it much easier for us to burn excess fat and maintain a healthy weight.

Immune function – Green Magic boosts immune function by providing the body with the nutritional building blocks our immune system needs and which are often not available in our normal diet in sufficient quantities for optimum immune function. Green Magic is particularly rich in B-complex vitamins, which are known to be very important for maintaining a healthy immune system.

Energy and vitality – Green Magic contains such a wide range of important nutrients that it can have a huge impact on people's energy and vitality levels. People who have unknowingly spent years surviving in a state of being "overfed and undernourished" suddenly feel transformed and alive when they give themselves the nutrients their bodies have been craving.

Detoxification – we've already mentioned the importance of detoxifying the body in the context of liver function and weight loss. Being able to detoxify the body is more important today than it has ever been, with so many pollutants, toxins and artificial chemicals in our environment – these are all poisons, many of which we are only beginning to understand in terms of the long-term damage they do to our bodies.

Digestion – again, we've already mentioned digestive health as it pertains to weight loss. However, digestive health is important for many other reasons too:

For example, getting the right kinds of soluble fibre in our diet improves cardiovascular health because it helps reduce the levels of bad (LDL) cholesterol in our bloodstream.

A compromised digestive system may lead, indirectly, to inflammation within the body and so increase our risk of suffering from a whole range of auto-immune diseases such as rheumatoid arthritis.

And of course, we need a healthy digestive system to be able to absorb all the macro- and micro-nutrients that our bodies need to stay healthy, maintain vitality and prevent disease. This is important at any age, but particularly so as we get older when digestion often becomes impaired.

Alkalising effects – the green superfoods in Green Magic produce what is known as an "alkaline ash" within the body, which is significant because – according to the American Dietetic Association – it may decrease the risk of osteoporosis.

While research remains ongoing, it also hypothesised that alkaline ash producing foods may help reduce the risk of heart disease, as well as increasing energy levels.

Oxygen free radicals – because it is so rich in vitamins, minerals, antioxidants and phyto-chemicals Green Magic has a powerful neutralising effect on dangerous oxygen free radicals.

Cardiovascular health – Green Magic improves cardiovascular health in a number of ways. We've already mentioned that the fibre and lecithin in Green Magic reduce bad (LDL) cholesterol levels in the bloodstream. The lecithin also emulsifies (breaks down) fats in the bloodstream, as well as helping us burn fat. In addition, the high levels of antioxidants and phyto-chemicals in Green Magic have a protective effect on our blood vessel linings, so helping to reduce the risk of arteriosclerosis.

Anti-aging – again, because of its ability to neutralise oxygen free radicals (a major cause of aging) Green Magic has powerful anti-aging properties. Plus, the high levels of micro-nutrients in Green Magic help to reduce the biological age of our cells – in other words it makes them younger.

In one study, carried out in the Ukraine at Kharkiv State University, scientists looked at the effect of Green Magic supplementation on biological age. The participants were divided into two groups. Those in the first group had calendar ages from 28 – 40; those in the second group had calendar ages from 41 – 65. The cellular biological age of the participants was measured at the start and at the end of the study.

Under clinical conditions the participants were given a serving of Green Magic every day for a total of three months.

At the end of the study the biological age of the first group (aged 28 – 40) had reduced by an average of 6 years. Meanwhile the biological age of the second, older, group (41 - 65) had reduced by an average of an incredible 13.5 years.

While this list covers the key health benefits of Green Magic it is by no means exhaustive. However, all of these things are vitally important for our health, vitality and energy levels as well as for long-term disease prevention.

How should you take Green Magic?

Green Magic is available in both powder and capsule form. Personally, I prefer the powder, but it makes absolutely no difference which you take. If you are taking Green Magic powder then it can be mixed in water, fruit or vegetable juice or even yoghurt.

Because it is made of whole-foods Green Magic can be taken at any time of day and on an empty stomach. I always like to take Green Magic first thing in the morning with breakfast. That way I know that I'm setting myself up for the day with some super high quality nutrition, as well as kicking the day off with the antioxidant equivalent of 5 servings of fruit and veg!

I then take a second serving of Green Magic in the afternoon and a third early evening to give myself further nutritional boosts as the day goes on.

If I am about to go for a run or work out I will time one of my three daily servings of Green Magic so that I take it just before I exercise. Exercise produces lots of dangerous oxygen free radicals. By having Green Magic *before* I exercise I know that I'm getting lots of antioxidants into my system that will help to neutralise these free radicals before they do serious harm.

Finally, if I'm feeling ill or run down (which happens much less now, since I've been taking Green Magic) I will take extra servings of Green Magic spaced throughout the day to boost my immune system.

For example, if I get that tickly throat feeling that can be the first sign of a cold what I have found is that I can often knock it on the head before it gets going by dosing up on Green Magic. What I'm actually doing it giving my immune system the building blocks and nutritional support it needs to ramp up quickly and fight the infection before it can get going. And even if it doesn't stop the cold completely it will reduce the severity and speed up my recovery time.

The 10/15 formula...

What all this means is that on a normal day I will take three servings of Green Magic – that's a lot of nutrition when combined with my daily fruit and veg intake!

This is where the 10/15 formula comes from:

Each day I aim for at least 10 servings of fruit and veg (that's where the 10 comes from) plus 3 servings of Green Magic. Each of those servings of Green Magic has the nutritional value of 5 servings of fruit and veg and so 3 x 5 gives us the 15.

Hence, we get the 10/15 formula, which gives us the nutritional equivalent of 25 servings per day.

The great thing about using the 10/15 formula to provide daily targets is that even if I fall a bit short I still know I'm getting massive amounts of high quality nutrition. For example, it's not always easy to hit 10 servings of fruit and veg in a day – especially when travelling. But even if I only hit half that number as long as I remember to take my Green Magic with me I can still hit 5/15 or the nutritional equivalent of 20 servings.

When you consider that the average person only manages around 3 servings a day it makes you realise what powerful nutritional support you are getting if you follow the 10/15 formula and get the equivalent of 25 servings per day. Suddenly you can begin to redress the balance – you can begin to compensate for all the damage that has been done to our food by intensive farming over the last 100 years, and through selection for taste over the last 10,000 years.

What are the next steps?

To enjoy the health and weight loss benefits that come from a healthy diet rich in fruit and veg and green superfoods you're going to need to take some action steps.

Step 1:

The first thing to do is to follow the 9 steps I set out earlier to start boosting the amount fruit and veg in your diet. Here's a quick reminder of what they are:

1) Go for variety
2) Convenience is crucial
3) Visibility is key
4) Every meal, every day
5) Snack on fruit, snack on veg
6) Half a plate... or more
7) If you're still feeling hungry keep going
8) Track your servings
9) Develop good habits

I recommend that you go back to the 9 steps and re-read them in full on a regular basis to begin with. This will help keep you on track and remind you of why they are important. Most of all, it will help with step 9, which is developing good habits. This is the most important step of all as once these things become habits they will become far easier to stick to – particularly over the long-term. You should aim to make all these things simply part of your normal lifestyle.

Step 2:

Step 2 is to incorporate green superfoods in your diet. Of all those on the market now the most complete and the most nutritious is, in my opinion, Green Magic. The biggest recommendation I can give you is to say that it's what I take; it's what I've taken for the last 19 years; *and, it's what I give to my family and recommend to friends.*

Like I said above, I recommend that you have a serving of Green Magic with your breakfast to start you day off right, followed by a second serving in the afternoon and a third in the evening for a total of three servings a day.

Again, developing the right habits around Green Magic is important. I recommend you keep it where you will see it and be reminded to take it with breakfast. Then set yourself a couple of reminders to take it during the day. Also, make sure you have it around when you when you need it – for example, keep some at work or take some with you when travelling.

If you can be really disciplined about taking Green Magic every day for the first week then you'll be well on the way to creating one of the most healthy and beneficial habits you'll ever develop!

Green Magic is available from a company called proto-col. To get Green Magic you need to visit this website where you'll be able to order it online:

https://www.proto-col.com/green-magic.html

Good luck and good health!

My congratulations to you for reading this book! I think it's awesome that you care about your health and are willing to take the necessary steps to transform it.

Keep it simple...

There's so much confusing and contradictory advice around on weight loss and what makes a healthy diet, but it's really not that complicated.

I've just given you two simple steps that will allow you to lose weight and optimise your nutrition:

Step 1: Get into the habit of eating plenty of fruit and veg – ideally 10 or more servings a day.

Step 2: Add a green superfood supplement like Green Magic to your diet to supercharge your nutrition intake and compensate for all the damage that's been done to the nutritional quality of our fruit and veg over the course of the last 10,000 years.

That's it – that's all you have to do!

To make Green Magic part of your life visit:
https://www.proto-col.com/green-magic.html

And while you're waiting for your Green Magic to arrive you can get down to your local supermarket or farmers' market and start stocking up on your favorite fruits and vegetables.

Then it's down to you to start building and strengthening those good habits.

All that remains now is for me to wish you good health and happiness!

About James Greenwell

JAMES GREENWELL is an entrepreneur, philanthropist and national champion athlete.

James competed for Great Britain as a Modern Pentathlete (running, swimming, shooting, fencing, show jumping) and during a sixteen year career earned over 50 international caps as well as becoming men's team captain.

Having gained a certificate in Nutrition and Diet with the International Therapy Council James launched his company, On Group Limited, in 2003 from his back bedroom in the city of Bath.

James first became interested in the role of nutrition for recovery following an injury that threatened to end his athletics career. His friend and modern pentathlon team mate Professor Greg Whyte OBE recommended collagen supplementation, which allowed James to make a dramatic recovery and a rapid return to athletics.

This sparked a deep fascination in nutrition for James and he has since built his business, On Group, to offer a wide range of nutritional supplements supporting sport performance, health and well-being. On Group products are now available in more than twenty countries and can be found on TV in the UK and France.

James continues to train and race as a Great Britain age group athlete and competes internationally in Biathle, Triathle and Aquathon. James lives in a village near Bath and loves to get out running local footpaths with friends and with his two cocker spaniel training partners, Wooster and Bingo.

www.ingramcontent.com/pod-product-compliance
Lightning Source LLC
Chambersburg PA
CBHW070621290526
45790CB00002B/946